I0781878

MATERNITY REFLEXOLOGY COMPENDIUM

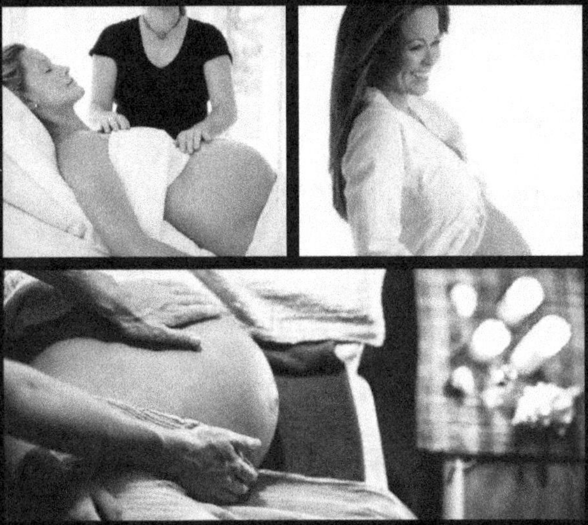

Dr. James K. Ferguson

COPYRIGHT © 2024 by Dr. James K. Ferguson

All rights reserved. No part of this publication may be reproduced, distributed, or transmitted in any form or by any means, including photocopying, recording, or other electronic or mechanical methods, without the prior written permission of the copyright owner, except in the case of brief quotations embodied in critical reviews and certain other noncommercial uses permitted by copyright law.

TABLE OF CONTENTS

TABLE OF CONTENTS ---------------------- 2-6

INTRODUCTION ------------------------------ 7-10

CHAPTER 1 ------------------------------------ 11-15

20 important things you should know about Maternity Reflexology

CHAPTER 2 ------------------------------------ 16-31

Overview of Maternity Reflexology: A Holistic Approach to Pregnancy Wellness

Benefits of Maternity Reflexology

How Maternity Reflexology Works

Safety Precautions and Guidelines

Benefits of Maternity Reflexology: Enhancing Pregnancy Wellness Naturally

How Maternity Reflexology Works: Understanding the Principles and Techniques

Techniques Used in Maternity Reflexology

Benefits of Maternity Reflexology During Pregnancy

Safety Precautions and Guidelines for Maternity Reflexology

CHAPTER 3 ------------------------------------ 32-38

Understanding Pregnancy: A Comprehensive Overview

How Pregnancy Affects the Body: A Comprehensive Guide

CHAPTER 4 ————————————————————— 39-53

Basics of Reflexology: Understanding the Principles and Benefits

Principles of Reflexology: Understanding the Foundation of Healing

How Reflexology Works: The Mechanisms of Healing

Benefits of Reflexology During Pregnancy: Supporting Maternal Health and Well-being

CHAPTER 5 ————————————————————— 54-69

Maternity Reflexology Techniques: Gentle and Effective Approaches for Pregnancy Wellness

Specific Reflexology Points for Pregnancy: Addressing Common Discomforts and Promoting Wellness

Special Considerations for Maternity Reflexology: Ensuring Safe and Effective Treatment

Combining Reflexology with Other Therapies: Enhancing Holistic Wellness

CHAPTER 6 ------------------------------------- 70-79

Reflexology for Common Pregnancy Issues

Reflexology for Nausea and Morning Sickness Relief During Pregnancy

Reflexology for Back Pain and Sciatica Relief During Pregnancy

CHAPTER 7 ------------------------------------- 80-86

Reflexology for Alleviating Swollen Ankles and Feet During Pregnancy

Reflexology for Improving Sleep and Alleviating Insomnia During Pregnancy

CHAPTER 8 ------------------------------------- 87-94

Reflexology for Labor Preparation: Supporting the Body's Natural Processes

Preparing for Labor with Reflexology: A Holistic Approach to Childbirth

CHAPTER 9 ------------------------------------- 95-102

Reflexology Techniques for Labor Induction: A Natural Approach to Stimulating Contractions

Reflexology for Pain Relief During Labor: Supporting Comfort and Relaxation

CHAPTER 10 ------------------------------------- 103-118

Postnatal Reflexology: Supporting Recovery and Well-being After Childbirth

Benefits of Postpartum Reflexology: Supporting Recovery and Well-being After Childbirth

Reflexology for Postpartum Recovery and Healing: Nurturing the Mother's Body and Mind

Reflexology for Postpartum Depression: Supporting Emotional Well-being

CHAPTER 11 ————————————————————— 119-133

Partner Reflexology Techniques and Support During Pregnancy

How Partners Can Support Each Other Through Reflexology During Pregnancy

Reflexology Techniques for Partners to Learn During Pregnancy

Reflexology for Bonding and Relaxation During Pregnancy

CHAPTER 12 ————————————————————— 134-149

Self-Care Reflexology Techniques for Pregnancy

Self-Reflexology Techniques for Pregnancy Wellness

Reflexology Techniques for Stress Relief and Relaxation

Reflexology for Emotional Well-being

CHAPTER 13 ———-------------------------------- 150-156

Summary of Key Points: Reflexology for Emotional Well-being

Glossary of Reflexology Terms

CONCLUSION ———-------------------------------- 157-160

INTRODUCTION

Pregnancy is a transformative journey filled with joy, anticipation, and a myriad of changes. As an expectant mother, you are embarking on a remarkable chapter of life, and it is natural to seek ways to enhance your well-being and the health of your baby. "Maternity Reflexology Compendium " is your comprehensive guide to utilizing the ancient art of reflexology to support and nurture you through every stage of pregnancy.

Understanding Pregnancy: The journey of pregnancy is a profound experience that encompasses physical, emotional, and spiritual changes. Each trimester brings its own set of challenges and milestones, from the initial excitement and adjustments of the first trimester to the physical changes and preparations for labor in the third trimester. Understanding these stages can help you navigate this journey with greater ease and confidence.

Benefits of Maternity Reflexology: Reflexology is a natural therapy that involves applying pressure to specific points on the feet, hands, or ears to stimulate healing and relaxation throughout the body. During pregnancy, reflexology can offer a range of benefits, including alleviating common discomforts such as nausea, back pain, and swollen ankles, as well as promoting relaxation and reducing stress.

How This Book Can Help You: "Maternity Reflexology Compendium " is designed to be your companion on this journey, providing you with practical techniques and insights to support your well-being and the health of your baby. Whether you are experiencing discomforts that come with pregnancy or simply seeking a way to relax and connect with your baby, this book offers a wealth of information to empower you to take charge of your health and wellness.

Safety Precautions and Guidelines: While reflexology is generally safe during pregnancy, it is important to practice it under the guidance of a trained professional. This book provides safety precautions and guidelines to ensure that you practice reflexology safely and effectively.

Pregnancy is a time of immense growth and transformation, both physically and emotionally. "Maternity Reflexology Compendium " is here to support you on this journey, offering you the knowledge and tools to enhance your well-being and nurture your connection with your baby. Whether you are seeking relief from pregnancy discomforts or simply looking for a way to relax and unwind, reflexology can be a valuable ally in your pregnancy toolkit.

CHAPTER 1

20 important things you should know about Maternity Reflexology

1. Maternity reflexology is a specialized form of reflexology tailored to the needs of pregnant women.

2. It focuses on specific points on the feet, hands, or ears that are believed to support pregnancy and childbirth.

3. Maternity reflexology can help reduce stress and anxiety during pregnancy, promoting a sense of well-being.

4. The therapy is safe and gentle, making it suitable for pregnant women at all stages of pregnancy.

5. It can help alleviate common pregnancy symptoms such as morning sickness, back pain, and swelling in the feet and ankles.

6. Maternity reflexology can also be beneficial during labor, helping to promote relaxation and manage pain.

7. The therapy is usually performed by a trained reflexologist who will tailor the treatment to the individual needs of the pregnant woman.

8. Maternity reflexology is often used as a complementary therapy alongside standard prenatal care.

9. It is important to consult with a healthcare provider before undergoing maternity reflexology, especially if you have any underlying health conditions or concerns.

10. Maternity reflexology can help promote a more comfortable and positive pregnancy experience.

11. The therapy is believed to work by stimulating the body's natural healing mechanisms and promoting balance and harmony within the body.

12. Maternity reflexology sessions are typically relaxing and enjoyable, providing a peaceful moment for the pregnant woman to connect with her body and her baby.

13. Some women may experience emotional releases during or after a maternity reflexology session, as the therapy can help release tension and promote relaxation.

14. Maternity reflexology can be beneficial for women who are struggling with fertility issues, as it can help promote relaxation and reduce stress levels.

15. The therapy can also be helpful for women postpartum, as it can help promote healing and balance in the body after childbirth.

16. Maternity reflexology is a holistic therapy that considers the physical, emotional, and spiritual aspects of pregnancy and childbirth.

17. It is important to choose a qualified and experienced reflexologist who has training in maternity reflexology.

18. Maternity reflexology is not a substitute for medical care, but it can be a valuable addition to a woman's prenatal and postnatal healthcare routine.

19. Some women may find that maternity reflexology helps them feel more connected to their baby during pregnancy, enhancing the bonding experience.

20. Overall, maternity reflexology is a gentle and effective therapy that can help support the health and well-being of both the pregnant woman and her baby.

CHAPTER 2

Overview of Maternity Reflexology: A Holistic Approach to Pregnancy Wellness

Maternity reflexology is a specialized form of reflexology that focuses on supporting and enhancing the well-being of expectant mothers throughout pregnancy. Rooted in the ancient practice of reflexology, which is based on the principle that specific points on the feet, hands, and ears correspond to different organs and systems in the body, maternity reflexology tailors these techniques to address the unique needs and changes experienced during pregnancy.

Benefits of Maternity Reflexology

One of the key benefits of maternity reflexology is its ability to provide natural relief for common pregnancy discomforts. By applying gentle pressure to specific reflex points, maternity reflexology can help alleviate issues such as morning sickness, back pain, swollen ankles, and insomnia. Additionally, maternity reflexology is known to promote relaxation and reduce stress, which can have a positive impact on both the mother and the developing baby.

How Maternity Reflexology Works

During pregnancy, the body undergoes a series of physiological and hormonal changes. These changes can sometimes lead to imbalances or discomforts. Maternity reflexology works by stimulating the reflex points associated with the reproductive system, as well as other relevant areas such as the endocrine system and the nervous system. By doing so, maternity reflexology can help restore balance and harmony to the body, promoting overall health and well-being.

Safety Precautions and Guidelines

While maternity reflexology is generally safe for most pregnant women, it is important to consult with a qualified reflexologist or healthcare provider before beginning any treatment. Certain reflex points, such as those associated with the uterus and ovaries, should be avoided during the first trimester to prevent the risk of miscarriage. Additionally, reflexologists should use gentle pressure and avoid vigorous techniques to ensure the safety of both the mother and the baby.

Maternity reflexology offers a safe, natural, and effective way to support the health and well-being of expectant mothers during pregnancy. By understanding the principles and benefits of maternity reflexology, mothers-to-be can empower themselves to take control of their health and enjoy a more comfortable and harmonious pregnancy journey. Whether used as a standalone therapy or as part of a comprehensive prenatal care plan, maternity reflexology has the potential to enhance the pregnancy experience and promote overall wellness for both mother and baby.

Benefits of Maternity Reflexology: Enhancing Pregnancy Wellness Naturally

Maternity reflexology offers a range of benefits for expectant mothers, providing a natural and holistic approach to pregnancy wellness.

Here are some key benefits:

1. Alleviation of Pregnancy Discomforts: Maternity reflexology can help alleviate common pregnancy discomforts such as nausea, back pain, swollen ankles, and fatigue. By targeting specific reflex points associated with these issues, reflexologists can help restore balance and provide relief.

2. Stress Reduction: Pregnancy can be a stressful time, both physically and emotionally.

Maternity reflexology promotes relaxation and helps reduce stress levels, which can have a positive impact on both the mother and the developing baby.

3. Improved Sleep: Many pregnant women struggle with insomnia and sleep disturbances. Maternity reflexology can help promote better sleep by relaxing the body and mind, making it easier to fall asleep and stay asleep.

4. Preparation for Labor: Reflexology can be used to prepare the body for labor by stimulating reflex points associated with the uterus and reproductive organs. This can help promote more efficient contractions and a smoother labor process.

5. Hormonal Balance: Pregnancy hormones can wreak havoc on the body, leading to mood swings, fatigue, and other issues. Maternity reflexology helps balance these hormones, promoting a sense of well-being and emotional stability.

6. Postnatal Recovery: Reflexology can also be beneficial during the postnatal period, helping the body recover from childbirth and promoting healing. It can help reduce swelling, relieve pain, and restore energy levels.

7. Bonding and Relaxation: Reflexology sessions can provide a peaceful and relaxing environment for mothers-to-be to bond with their unborn babies. It can be a time for reflection, connection, and nurturing the mother-child relationship.

8. Complementary Therapy: Maternity reflexology can be used as a complementary therapy alongside conventional prenatal care. It is non-invasive and safe, making it a popular choice for pregnant women looking for natural ways to enhance their pregnancy experience.

In summary, maternity reflexology offers a range of benefits for expectant mothers, providing a natural and holistic approach to pregnancy wellness. Whether used to alleviate discomforts, reduce stress, or prepare for labor, reflexology can be a valuable tool in promoting a healthy and happy pregnancy journey.

How Maternity Reflexology Works: Understanding the Principles and Techniques

Maternity reflexology is based on the principle that certain reflex points on the feet, hands, and ears correspond to specific organs and systems in the body. By applying pressure to these reflex points, a reflexologist can stimulate the body's natural healing processes and promote overall wellness.

During pregnancy, a woman's body undergoes a series of changes, both physical and hormonal. Maternity reflexology aims to support these changes by focusing on reflex points that are particularly relevant to pregnancy and childbirth.

Techniques Used in Maternity Reflexology

1. Gentle Pressure: Reflexologists use their hands to apply gentle pressure to specific reflex points. The pressure should be firm but not painful, and the technique is often described as relaxing and soothing.

2. Thumb Walking: This technique involves using the thumbs to walk along the reflex points, applying pressure in a rhythmic and methodical manner. Thumb walking helps to stimulate the reflex points and promote relaxation.

3. Rotation: Reflexologists may also use a rotating motion on certain reflex points to help release tension and improve circulation.

4. Massage: In addition to working on the reflex points, reflexologists may incorporate massage techniques to further relax the body and promote a sense of well-being.

Benefits of Maternity Reflexology During Pregnancy

1. Alleviation of Discomforts: By targeting specific reflex points, maternity reflexology can help alleviate common pregnancy discomforts such as nausea, back pain, and swollen ankles.

2. Stress Reduction: Reflexology promotes relaxation and reduces stress levels, which can be beneficial for both the mother and the baby.

3. Preparation for Labor: Reflexology can help prepare the body for labor by stimulating reflex points associated with the uterus and reproductive organs.

4. Hormonal Balance: Reflexology helps balance hormones, promoting emotional well-being and stability during pregnancy.

5. Improved Sleep: Many pregnant women experience insomnia and sleep disturbances, and reflexology can help promote better sleep patterns.

In summary, maternity reflexology works by stimulating specific reflex points on the feet, hands, and ears to promote relaxation, alleviate discomforts, and support overall wellness during pregnancy. It is a safe and natural therapy that can be a valuable addition to prenatal care.

Safety Precautions and Guidelines for Maternity Reflexology

While maternity reflexology is generally safe for most pregnant women, it is important to take certain precautions to ensure the safety and well-being of both the mother and the baby.

Here are some safety precautions and guidelines to keep in mind:

1. Consultation with Healthcare Provider: Before beginning maternity reflexology, it is advisable to consult with your healthcare provider, especially if you have any underlying health conditions or complications with your pregnancy.

2. Qualified Reflexologist: Ensure that your reflexologist is qualified and experienced in providing maternity reflexology. They should be knowledgeable about the specific reflex points to avoid or focus on during pregnancy.

3. Avoid Certain Reflex Points: During the first trimester, it is recommended to avoid certain reflex points associated with the uterus and ovaries to reduce the risk of miscarriage. A qualified reflexologist will know which points to avoid and will adjust the treatment accordingly.

4. Gentle Pressure: Reflexologists should use gentle pressure and avoid any vigorous or deep tissue techniques, as this can be harmful during pregnancy.

5. Communication: It is important to communicate openly with your reflexologist about any discomfort or pain you may experience during the treatment. They can adjust the pressure and techniques accordingly.

6. Hydration: Drink plenty of water before and after the treatment to stay hydrated and help flush out toxins released during the reflexology session.

7. Comfortable Position: Ensure that you are in a comfortable position during the reflexology session, either sitting or lying down, with support for your back and legs if needed.

8. Frequency of Sessions: While maternity reflexology can be beneficial, it is recommended to limit the frequency of sessions, especially in the first trimester. Your reflexologist can advise you on the appropriate frequency based on your individual needs.

9. Monitoring: After the reflexology session, monitor how you feel and report any unusual symptoms to your healthcare provider.

In summary, maternity reflexology can be a safe and effective way to support your pregnancy wellness, but it is important to take precautions and follow guidelines to ensure a safe and beneficial experience for you and your baby. Always consult with your healthcare provider before beginning any new therapy during pregnancy.

CHAPTER 3

Understanding Pregnancy: A Comprehensive Overview

Pregnancy is a transformative journey that involves a series of physiological and hormonal changes in a woman's body as it prepares for childbirth. Understanding these changes is key to navigating pregnancy with knowledge and confidence.

Stages of Pregnancy: Pregnancy is typically divided into three trimesters, each lasting about three months. The first trimester is characterized by rapid changes as the fertilized egg implants in the uterus and begins to develop into a fetus. The second trimester is often referred to as the "honeymoon period" as many women experience a reduction in symptoms such as morning sickness. The third trimester is marked by further fetal development and preparation for childbirth.

Common Pregnancy Discomforts: Pregnancy can bring about a range of discomforts, including morning sickness, fatigue, back pain, and swollen ankles. These discomforts are often a result of hormonal changes and the physical strain of carrying a growing baby.

Impact on the Body: Pregnancy has a profound impact on a woman's body, affecting nearly every system, including the cardiovascular, respiratory, and digestive systems. Hormonal changes play a key role in these adaptations, preparing the body for childbirth and breastfeeding.

Emotional Changes: Pregnancy is also a time of emotional changes, as women experience a range of feelings from joy and excitement to anxiety and mood swings. Hormonal fluctuations, coupled with the stress of preparing for a new arrival, can contribute to these emotional changes.

Preparation for Labor: As pregnancy progresses, the body begins to prepare for labor and childbirth. This includes physical changes such as the softening of the cervix and the positioning of the baby in the pelvis. Women may also experience Braxton Hicks contractions, which are practice contractions that help prepare the uterus for labor.

Understanding pregnancy is essential for expectant mothers to navigate this journey with confidence and knowledge. By understanding the stages of pregnancy, common discomforts, and the impact on the body, women can better prepare themselves for the physical and emotional changes that come with pregnancy. It is important for women to seek regular prenatal care and consult with healthcare providers for personalized guidance and support throughout their pregnancy journey.

How Pregnancy Affects the Body: A Comprehensive Guide

Pregnancy is a transformative experience that affects nearly every aspect of a woman's body. From hormonal changes to physical adaptations, understanding how pregnancy impacts the body is crucial for expectant mothers.

Hormonal Changes: During pregnancy, the body experiences a surge in hormones, including estrogen and progesterone, which play a crucial role in maintaining the pregnancy and preparing the body for childbirth. These hormonal changes can lead to a variety of symptoms, including morning sickness, mood swings, and changes in skin pigmentation.

Physical Adaptations: As the baby grows, the uterus expands to accommodate the growing fetus. This can lead to physical changes such as weight gain, changes in posture, and a shifting center of gravity. The increased weight and pressure on the pelvis can also lead to back pain and discomfort.

Cardiovascular System: Pregnancy places increased demands on the cardiovascular system, as the body needs to supply more blood to the uterus and placenta. This can lead to an increase in blood volume and heart rate, as well as changes in blood pressure.

Respiratory System: The growing uterus can also put pressure on the diaphragm, leading to shortness of breath and difficulty breathing, especially in the later stages of pregnancy.

Digestive System: Pregnancy can also affect the digestive system, leading to symptoms such as constipation, bloating, and heartburn. These symptoms are often a result of hormonal changes and the pressure of the growing uterus on the digestive organs.

Musculoskeletal System: The hormone relaxin, which is released during pregnancy, helps relax the ligaments in the pelvis to prepare for childbirth. However, it can also affect other joints in the body, leading to increased flexibility and a higher risk of injury.

Pregnancy is a complex and dynamic process that affects the body in numerous ways. By understanding how pregnancy impacts the body, expectant mothers can better prepare themselves for the physical changes and challenges that come with pregnancy. Seeking regular prenatal care and consulting with healthcare providers can help ensure a healthy pregnancy and delivery.

CHAPTER 4

Basics of Reflexology: Understanding the Principles and Benefits

Reflexology is an ancient healing practice that involves applying pressure to specific points on the feet, hands, or ears to stimulate a healing response in corresponding organs and systems of the body.

Here are the basics of reflexology:

1. Principles of Reflexology: Reflexology is based on the principle that there are reflex points on the feet, hands, and ears that correspond to specific organs, glands, and other parts of the body. By applying pressure to these reflex points, a reflexologist can help stimulate energy flow and promote healing in the corresponding areas of the body.

2. Benefits of Reflexology: Reflexology offers a range of benefits, including stress reduction, relaxation, improved circulation, and pain relief. It is often used to treat conditions such as headaches, digestive disorders, and hormonal imbalances. Reflexology is also commonly used to promote overall health and well-being.

3. Techniques Used in Reflexology: Reflexologists use their hands to apply pressure to specific reflex points on the feet, hands, or ears. The pressure should be firm but not painful, and the techniques are often described as relaxing and soothing. Reflexologists may also use thumb walking, rotation, and massage techniques to stimulate the reflex points.

4. Safety Precautions: While reflexology is generally safe for most people, there are some precautions to keep in mind. Pregnant women, individuals with certain medical conditions, and those with foot injuries or infections should consult with a healthcare provider before undergoing reflexology.

5. Reflexology Sessions: A typical reflexology session lasts about 30 to 60 minutes. During the session, the reflexologist will work on specific reflex points on the feet, hands, or ears, depending on the client's needs. Clients often report feeling deeply relaxed and rejuvenated after a reflexology session.

6. Integrative Approach: Reflexology is often used as part of an integrative healthcare approach, complementing other treatments such as massage therapy, acupuncture, and chiropractic care. It is believed that reflexology can help enhance the effectiveness of these other treatments and promote overall health and wellness.

In summary, reflexology is a holistic healing practice that offers a range of benefits for the body and mind. By understanding the basics of reflexology, individuals can explore this ancient healing art as a way to promote health, relaxation, and overall well-being.

Principles of Reflexology: Understanding the Foundation of Healing

Reflexology is based on several key principles that guide its practice and effectiveness. These principles form the foundation of reflexology's holistic approach to healing and well-being. **Here are the key principles of reflexology:**

1. Reflex Zones: Reflexology is based on the concept that the body is divided into ten longitudinal zones, with each zone corresponding to specific areas of the body, including organs, glands, and other body parts. By applying pressure to specific points within these zones, a reflexologist can help stimulate healing and relaxation in the corresponding areas of the body.

2. Reflex Points: Within each reflex zone are reflex points that correspond to specific organs, glands, and other body parts. These reflex points are located on the feet, hands, and ears, and by applying pressure to these points, a reflexologist can help stimulate energy flow and promote healing in the corresponding areas of the body.

3. Energy Flow: Reflexology is based on the belief that there is a vital energy, or life force, that flows through the body along specific pathways known as meridians. By applying pressure to specific reflex points, a reflexologist can help restore the flow of energy along these meridians, promoting health and well-being.

4. Healing Response: Reflexology stimulates the body's natural healing mechanisms, encouraging the body to heal itself. By applying pressure to specific reflex points, reflexologists can help trigger a healing response in the corresponding areas of the body, promoting relaxation, pain relief, and overall well-being.

5. Holistic Approach: Reflexology takes a holistic approach to healing, treating the body, mind, and spirit as interconnected parts of a whole. By addressing imbalances in the body's energy flow, reflexology can help restore balance and promote health and well-being on all levels.

6. Individualized Treatment: Reflexology recognizes that each person is unique, and as such, treatments are tailored to the individual's specific needs and health goals. Reflexologists work with clients to identify areas of imbalance and develop a treatment plan that addresses these imbalances to promote healing and well-being.

In summary, the principles of reflexology are based on the idea that the body has the ability to heal itself, and by stimulating specific reflex points, a reflexologist can help facilitate this healing process. Reflexology takes a holistic approach to healing, addressing the body, mind, and spirit to promote health and well-being on all levels.

How Reflexology Works: The Mechanisms of Healing

Reflexology works on the principle that there are reflex points on the feet, hands, and ears that correspond to specific organs, glands, and other parts of the body. By applying pressure to these reflex points, a reflexologist can help stimulate energy flow and promote healing in the corresponding areas of the body.

Here's how reflexology works:

1. Nerve Stimulation: When pressure is applied to a reflex point, it stimulates the nerve endings in that area. These nerves then send signals to the brain, which in turn sends signals to the corresponding body part. This stimulation helps to improve nerve function and communication within the body.

2. Blood Circulation: Reflexology helps to improve blood circulation throughout the body. By stimulating reflex points, reflexologists can help dilate blood vessels, which allows for better blood flow to organs and tissues. Improved circulation can help promote healing and reduce inflammation.

3. Relaxation Response: Reflexology promotes relaxation by activating the parasympathetic nervous system, which is responsible for rest and relaxation. This can help reduce stress, tension, and anxiety, and promote a sense of well-being.

4. Toxin Removal: Reflexology can help stimulate the lymphatic system, which is responsible for removing toxins and waste products from the body. By improving lymphatic drainage, reflexology can help detoxify the body and improve overall health.

5. Energy Flow: According to traditional Chinese medicine, reflexology helps to balance the flow of energy, or Qi, throughout the body.

By stimulating reflex points, reflexologists can help remove blockages in the energy pathways, promoting health and well-being.

6. Pain Relief: Reflexology can help reduce pain by stimulating the release of endorphins, which are natural painkillers produced by the body. By activating the body's natural pain relief mechanisms, reflexology can help alleviate pain and discomfort.

In summary, reflexology works by stimulating specific reflex points on the feet, hands, or ears to promote healing and well-being in the corresponding areas of the body. By improving nerve function, increasing blood circulation, promoting relaxation, and removing toxins, reflexology can help restore balance and promote health on all levels.

Benefits of Reflexology During Pregnancy: Supporting Maternal Health and Well-being

Reflexology offers a range of benefits for expectant mothers, providing a safe and natural way to support maternal health and well-being throughout pregnancy.

Here are some key benefits of reflexology during pregnancy:

1. Stress Reduction: Pregnancy can be a stressful time, both physically and emotionally. Reflexology helps to promote relaxation and reduce stress levels, which can benefit both the mother and the developing baby.

2. Pain Relief: Many pregnant women experience aches and pains, particularly in the lower back, hips, and legs. Reflexology can help alleviate these discomforts by promoting relaxation and reducing muscle tension.

3. Improved Sleep: Sleep disturbances are common during pregnancy, but reflexology can help promote better sleep patterns by inducing a state of deep relaxation.

4. Hormonal Balance: Pregnancy hormones can lead to mood swings and other emotional imbalances. Reflexology helps to balance these hormones, promoting emotional well-being and stability.

5. Preparation for Labor: Reflexology can help prepare the body for labor by stimulating reflex points associated with the reproductive organs. This can help promote more efficient contractions and a smoother labor process.

6. Reduced Swelling: Many pregnant women experience swelling, particularly in the feet and ankles. Reflexology can help reduce swelling by improving circulation and lymphatic drainage.

7. Immune Support: Reflexology helps to stimulate the body's natural healing processes, which can support the immune system and help prevent illness during pregnancy.

8. Bonding: Reflexology sessions can provide a peaceful and nurturing environment for mothers-to-be to bond with their unborn babies. It can be a time for relaxation, reflection, and connection.

In summary, reflexology offers a range of benefits for expectant mothers, providing a safe and natural way to support maternal health and well-being during pregnancy. By promoting relaxation, reducing stress, alleviating pain, and supporting overall health, reflexology can help mothers-to-be enjoy a more comfortable and harmonious pregnancy journey.

CHAPTER 5

Maternity Reflexology Techniques: Gentle and Effective Approaches for Pregnancy Wellness

Maternity reflexology involves the application of gentle pressure to specific reflex points on the feet, hands, or ears to support the health and well-being of expectant mothers.

Here are some key techniques used in maternity reflexology:

1. Thumb Walking: This technique involves using the thumbs to walk along the reflex points on the feet. The reflexologist applies gentle pressure to each point, moving in a systematic and rhythmic manner. Thumb walking helps to stimulate the reflex points and promote relaxation.

2. Rotation: Reflexologists may use a rotating motion on certain reflex points to help release tension and improve circulation. This technique can help to promote the flow of energy and enhance the body's natural healing processes.

3. Gentle Pressure: Maternity reflexology uses gentle pressure to avoid causing discomfort or pain. The pressure should be firm but not painful, and the reflexologist should always check in with the client to ensure they are comfortable.

4. Focus on Specific Points: During pregnancy, there are certain reflex points that are particularly beneficial to stimulate. These include points associated with the reproductive organs, such as the ovaries and uterus, as well as points that can help alleviate common pregnancy discomforts, such as nausea and back pain.

5. Use of Essential Oils: Some reflexologists may use essential oils during maternity reflexology sessions to enhance the therapeutic effects. Essential oils such as lavender or chamomile can help promote relaxation and reduce stress.

6. Hand and Ear Reflexology: In addition to the feet, reflexologists may also work on the hands and ears during maternity reflexology sessions. The hands and ears contain reflex points that correspond to different parts of the body, and stimulating these points can help promote overall health and well-being.

7. Tailored Approach: Maternity reflexology is tailored to the individual needs of each client. Reflexologists will take into account the client's specific symptoms, concerns, and stage of pregnancy when developing a treatment plan.

In summary, maternity reflexology uses gentle and effective techniques to support the health and well-being of expectant mothers. By stimulating specific reflex points, reflexologists can help alleviate common pregnancy discomforts, promote relaxation, and enhance the overall pregnancy experience.

Specific Reflexology Points for Pregnancy: Addressing Common Discomforts and Promoting Wellness

Reflexology during pregnancy focuses on specific reflex points that can help alleviate common discomforts and promote overall wellness for expectant mothers.

Here are some key reflex points that are often targeted during maternity reflexology sessions:

1. Pituitary Gland (Big Toe): Stimulating the reflex point for the pituitary gland, located on the big toe, can help regulate hormone levels and promote hormonal balance during pregnancy.

2. Uterus (Heel): The reflex point for the uterus is located on the heel of the foot. Stimulating this point can help promote healthy uterine function and support the body during pregnancy.

3. Ovaries (Outer Foot): The reflex points for the ovaries are located on the outer edge of the foot, near the ankle. Stimulating these points can help support hormonal balance and reproductive health during pregnancy.

4. Kidneys (Inner Foot): The reflex points for the kidneys are located on the inner edge of the foot, near the arch. Stimulating these points can help promote kidney function and reduce fluid retention, a common issue during pregnancy.

5. Digestive System (Ball of Foot): The reflex points for the digestive system are located on the ball of the foot, near the base of the toes. Stimulating these points can help alleviate digestive issues such as nausea, indigestion, and constipation.

6. Pelvic Area (Lower Foot): The reflex points for the pelvic area are located on the lower part of the foot, near the heel. Stimulating these points can help promote pelvic health and support the body as it prepares for childbirth.

7. Adrenal Glands (Top of Foot): The reflex points for the adrenal glands are located on the top of the foot, near the ankle. Stimulating these points can help support the body's stress response and promote relaxation during pregnancy.

8. Solar Plexus (Center of Foot): The reflex point for the solar plexus, a complex network of nerves in the abdomen, is located in the center of the foot. Stimulating this point can help promote relaxation and reduce stress and anxiety during pregnancy.

In summary, reflexology during pregnancy targets specific reflex points to help alleviate common discomforts and promote overall wellness for expectant mothers. By stimulating these points, reflexologists can help support the body's natural healing processes and enhance the pregnancy experience.

Special Considerations for Maternity Reflexology: Ensuring Safe and Effective Treatment

Maternity reflexology requires special considerations to ensure the safety and well-being of both the mother and the baby. Reflexologists must take into account the unique needs and concerns of pregnant women when performing reflexology treatments.

Here are some key considerations for maternity reflexology:

1. **Trimester-Specific Techniques:** Reflexologists should tailor their techniques based on the stage of pregnancy. For example, during the first trimester, it is important to avoid stimulating certain reflex points associated with the reproductive organs to reduce the risk of

miscarriage. Reflexologists should also use lighter pressure and avoid deep tissue techniques throughout pregnancy.

2. Positioning: Pregnant women may be uncomfortable lying flat on their backs for extended periods, especially in the later stages of pregnancy. Reflexologists should offer pillows or cushions to support the mother's back and ensure she is comfortable during the treatment. Some reflexologists may also offer reflexology in a seated position for added comfort.

3. Avoiding Certain Reflex Points: Reflexologists should avoid stimulating reflex points associated with the pituitary gland, ovaries, and uterus during the first trimester to reduce the risk of miscarriage. Additionally, reflexologists should avoid strong pressure on the ankle and calf reflex points to reduce the risk of blood clots.

4. Communication: Open communication between the reflexologist and the client is essential during maternity reflexology. Pregnant women should inform their reflexologist about any pregnancy-related symptoms or concerns they may have so that the treatment can be tailored to their individual needs.

5. Hydration: Pregnant women should be encouraged to drink plenty of water before and after the reflexology treatment to stay hydrated and help flush out toxins released during the session.

6. Frequency of Treatments: While reflexology can be beneficial during pregnancy, it is recommended to limit the frequency of treatments, especially in the first trimester. Reflexologists should work with pregnant clients to develop a treatment plan that is safe and appropriate for their individual needs.

7. Consultation with Healthcare Provider: Pregnant women should consult with their healthcare provider before undergoing reflexology treatment, especially if they have any underlying health conditions or complications with their pregnancy.

In summary, maternity reflexology requires special considerations to ensure the safety and well-being of pregnant women. Reflexologists should tailor their techniques, positioning, and treatment plans to meet the unique needs of pregnant clients and promote a safe and effective treatment experience.

Combining Reflexology with Other Therapies: Enhancing Holistic Wellness

Combining reflexology with other complementary therapies can enhance the overall wellness experience and provide a more comprehensive approach to healing.

Here are some common therapies that can be combined with reflexology:

1. Aromatherapy: Aromatherapy involves the use of essential oils to promote health and well-being. By combining aromatherapy with reflexology, the therapeutic effects of both modalities can be enhanced. For example, lavender essential oil can promote relaxation and reduce stress when used in conjunction with reflexology.

2. Massage Therapy: Massage therapy and reflexology both focus on promoting relaxation and reducing tension in the body. Combining the two therapies can provide a more comprehensive approach to relieving muscle tension and promoting overall relaxation.

3. Acupuncture: Acupuncture is a traditional Chinese medicine practice that involves the insertion of thin needles into specific points on the body to promote healing and relieve pain. When combined with reflexology, acupuncture can help enhance the flow of energy throughout the body and promote overall balance and wellness.

4. Reiki: Reiki is a form of energy healing that involves the practitioner channeling universal energy to promote healing and relaxation. Combining Reiki with reflexology can help enhance the body's natural healing processes and promote a deeper sense of relaxation and well-being.

5. Yoga: Yoga is a holistic practice that combines physical postures, breathing exercises, and meditation to promote health and well-being. When combined with reflexology, yoga can help enhance the overall relaxation and stress-relief benefits of both practices.

6. Chiropractic Care: Chiropractic care focuses on the alignment of the spine and nervous system to promote health and wellness. When combined with reflexology, chiropractic care can help promote overall balance and alignment in the body, enhancing the effectiveness of both therapies.

7. Nutrition and Lifestyle Counseling: Good nutrition and healthy lifestyle habits are essential for overall health and well-being. Combining reflexology with nutrition and lifestyle counseling can help clients make positive changes in their diet and lifestyle to support their overall wellness goals.

In summary, combining reflexology with other complementary therapies can enhance the overall wellness experience and provide a more holistic approach to healing. By integrating these therapies, individuals can address the physical, emotional, and spiritual aspects of their health and well-being, promoting a more balanced and harmonious life.

CHAPTER 6

Reflexology for Common Pregnancy Issues

Reflexology can be a safe and effective complementary therapy to help alleviate common pregnancy issues.

Here's how reflexology can help with some of these issues:

1. Morning Sickness: Reflexology can help relieve nausea and vomiting associated with morning sickness by stimulating the reflex points for the stomach and digestive system. This can help improve digestion and reduce feelings of nausea.

2. Back Pain: Pregnancy often leads to back pain due to the extra weight and changes in posture. Reflexology can help relieve back pain by stimulating reflex points associated with the spine and muscles of the back, promoting relaxation and reducing tension.

3. Edema (Swelling): Many pregnant women experience swelling, particularly in the feet and ankles. Reflexology can help reduce swelling by improving circulation and lymphatic drainage, helping to remove excess fluid from the body.

4. Insomnia: Sleep disturbances are common during pregnancy, but reflexology can help promote better sleep patterns by inducing a state of deep relaxation and reducing stress and anxiety.

5. Fatigue: Pregnancy can be physically and emotionally draining, leading to fatigue. Reflexology can help reduce fatigue by stimulating reflex points associated with energy levels and promoting relaxation.

6. Hormonal Imbalances: Pregnancy hormones can lead to mood swings and other emotional imbalances. Reflexology can help balance hormones by stimulating the pituitary gland and other endocrine glands, promoting emotional well-being and stability.

7. Preparation for Labor: Reflexology can help prepare the body for labor by stimulating reflex points associated with the reproductive organs and promoting relaxation. This can help promote more efficient contractions and a smoother labor process.

8. General Relaxation and Stress Relief: Pregnancy can be a stressful time, but reflexology can help promote relaxation and reduce stress levels. This can benefit both the mother and the developing baby.

It's important to note that while reflexology can be a beneficial therapy during pregnancy, it should always be done by a qualified reflexologist who has experience working with pregnant women. Pregnant women should also consult with their healthcare provider before undergoing reflexology or any other complementary therapy.

Reflexology for Nausea and Morning Sickness Relief During Pregnancy

Nausea and morning sickness are common discomforts experienced by many pregnant women, especially in the first trimester. Reflexology can be a safe and effective complementary therapy to help alleviate these symptoms.

Here's how reflexology can help:

1. Stomach Reflex Point: The reflex point for the stomach is located on the ball of the foot, near the base of the toes. By applying gentle pressure to this point, reflexologists can help stimulate digestion and reduce feelings of nausea.

2. Diaphragm Reflex Point: The diaphragm reflex point is located just below the ball of the foot, in the center. Stimulating this point can help relax the diaphragm and promote deeper breathing, which can help reduce feelings of nausea.

3. Solar Plexus Reflex Point: The solar plexus is a complex network of nerves in the abdomen that is associated with the digestive system. The reflex point for the solar plexus is located in the center of the foot. Stimulating this point can help promote relaxation and reduce stress, which can help alleviate nausea.

4. Liver Reflex Point: The liver plays a role in digestion and detoxification, and stimulating the liver reflex point, located on the right foot, can help support liver function and reduce nausea.

5. Kidney Reflex Point: The kidneys are responsible for filtering waste products from the blood, and stimulating the kidney reflex points, located on the inner edge of the foot, near the arch, can help promote detoxification and reduce nausea.

Reflexology sessions for nausea and morning sickness are typically gentle and relaxing. It's important for pregnant women to communicate with their reflexologist about their symptoms and comfort levels during the session. Pregnant women should also consult with their healthcare provider before undergoing reflexology or any other complementary therapy.

Reflexology for Back Pain and Sciatica Relief During Pregnancy

Back pain and sciatica are common issues experienced by many pregnant women due to the changes in their body's structure and the increased strain on the back muscles. Reflexology can be a supportive therapy to help alleviate these discomforts.

Here's how reflexology can help:

1. Spine Reflex Points: Reflexologists focus on stimulating reflex points along the spine on the feet, which correspond to the vertebrae and muscles of the back. By applying gentle pressure to these points, reflexologists can help relieve tension and promote relaxation in the back muscles.

2. Sciatic Nerve Reflex Points: The sciatic nerve is the largest nerve in the body and can become compressed during pregnancy, leading to sciatica. Reflexologists can stimulate reflex points on the feet that correspond to the sciatic nerve to help alleviate pain and discomfort.

3. Pelvic Reflex Points: The pelvis undergoes significant changes during pregnancy, which can contribute to back pain. Reflexologists can target reflex points on the feet that correspond to the pelvis to help relieve tension and promote relaxation in this area.

4. Kidney Reflex Points: The kidneys play a role in the body's ability to eliminate waste products and maintain fluid balance. Reflexologists can stimulate kidney reflex points on the feet to help reduce fluid retention, which can contribute to back pain and sciatica.

5. General Relaxation: Reflexology promotes relaxation and can help reduce stress, which can exacerbate back pain. By inducing a state of deep relaxation, reflexologists can help alleviate muscle tension and promote overall well-being.

Reflexology sessions for back pain and sciatica are tailored to the individual needs of the client and are typically gentle and relaxing. Pregnant women should communicate with their reflexologist about their symptoms and comfort levels during the session. It's also important for pregnant women to consult with their healthcare provider before undergoing reflexology or any other complementary therapy.

CHAPTER 7

Reflexology for Alleviating Swollen Ankles and Feet During Pregnancy

Swelling, especially in the ankles and feet, is a common discomfort experienced by many pregnant women due to increased pressure on the veins and the body's retention of fluids. Reflexology can be a supportive therapy to help reduce swelling and promote overall comfort. **Here's how reflexology can help:**

1. Lymphatic System Stimulation: Reflexologists can stimulate reflex points on the feet that correspond to the lymphatic system, which helps the body remove excess fluid and waste. By promoting lymphatic drainage, reflexology can help reduce swelling in the ankles and feet.

2. Kidney Reflex Points: The kidneys play a key role in regulating fluid balance in the body. Reflexologists can stimulate reflex points on the feet that correspond to the kidneys to help promote kidney function and reduce fluid retention.

3. Circulation Improvement: Reflexology can help improve blood circulation, which can reduce swelling in the ankles and feet. By stimulating reflex points associated with circulation, reflexologists can help promote the flow of blood and lymphatic fluid, reducing fluid buildup.

4.   Relaxation   and   Stress   Reduction:
Reflexology promotes relaxation and can help reduce stress, which can contribute to fluid retention. By inducing a state of deep relaxation, reflexologists can help alleviate tension and promote overall well-being.

5. General Foot and Ankle Reflex Points:
Reflexologists can target reflex points on the feet and ankles that correspond to these areas. By applying gentle pressure to these points, reflexologists can help reduce swelling and promote comfort.

Reflexology sessions for swollen ankles and feet are typically gentle and focused on promoting relaxation and circulation. Pregnant women should communicate with their reflexologist about their symptoms and comfort levels during the session. It's also important for pregnant women to consult with their healthcare provider before undergoing reflexology or any other complementary therapy.

Reflexology for Improving Sleep and Alleviating Insomnia During Pregnancy

Insomnia and sleep issues are common concerns for many pregnant women, particularly in the later stages of pregnancy. Reflexology can be a helpful complementary therapy to promote relaxation and improve sleep quality.

Here's how reflexology can help:

1. Relaxation Response: Reflexology promotes relaxation by activating the parasympathetic nervous system, which is responsible for rest and relaxation. By inducing a state of deep relaxation, reflexologists can help reduce stress and anxiety, making it easier to fall asleep.

2. Hormonal Balance: Reflexology helps to balance hormones, including melatonin, which is responsible for regulating sleep-wake cycles. By stimulating reflex points associated with hormonal balance, reflexologists can help improve sleep patterns.

3. Stress Reduction: Reflexology helps to reduce stress, which can be a major contributing factor to insomnia. By promoting relaxation and reducing tension, reflexologists can help calm the mind and body, making it easier to achieve restful sleep.

4. General Relaxation: Reflexology promotes overall relaxation, which can help prepare the body for sleep. By releasing tension in the muscles and promoting a sense of calm, reflexologists can help improve sleep quality.

5. Circulation Improvement: Reflexology can help improve blood circulation, which can help promote relaxation and reduce restlessness. By stimulating reflex points associated with circulation, reflexologists can help improve overall sleep quality.

6. Endorphin Release: Reflexology stimulates the release of endorphins, which are natural painkillers and mood enhancers. By promoting the release of endorphins, reflexologists can help reduce pain and promote feelings of well-being, which can contribute to better sleep.

Reflexology sessions for insomnia and sleep issues are typically gentle and focused on promoting relaxation. Pregnant women should communicate with their reflexologist about their symptoms and comfort levels during the session. It's also important for pregnant women to consult with their healthcare provider before undergoing reflexology or any other complementary therapy.

CHAPTER 8

Reflexology for Labor Preparation: Supporting the Body's Natural Processes

Reflexology can be a valuable tool to help prepare the body for labor and childbirth. By stimulating specific reflex points on the feet, hands, or ears, reflexology can help promote relaxation, balance hormones, and support overall well-being, which can be beneficial during labor.

Here's how reflexology can help with labor preparation:

1. Uterus and Pelvic Reflex Points: Reflexologists target reflex points that correspond to the uterus and pelvic area to help promote uterine contractions and prepare the body for labor. Stimulating these points can help support the natural progression of labor.

2. Hormonal Balance: Reflexology helps to balance hormones, including oxytocin, which is known as the "love hormone" and plays a key role in childbirth. By stimulating reflex points associated with hormonal balance, reflexologists can help support the body's natural processes during labor.

3. Pain Relief: Reflexology can help alleviate pain and discomfort during labor by stimulating reflex points associated with pain relief. This can help women cope with the intensity of contractions and promote a more comfortable labor experience.

4. Relaxation: Reflexology promotes relaxation and reduces stress, which can be beneficial during labor. By inducing a state of deep relaxation, reflexologists can help women remain calm and focused during labor.

5. Energy Balance: Reflexology helps to balance the body's energy levels, which can be important during labor. By stimulating reflex points associated with energy levels, reflexologists can help women maintain their stamina and endurance during labor.

6. Mental Preparation: Reflexology can help women mentally prepare for labor by promoting a sense of calm and reducing anxiety. By stimulating reflex points associated with relaxation and mental clarity, reflexologists can help women feel more confident and prepared for labor.

Overall, reflexology can be a valuable tool to help prepare the body for labor and childbirth. It is important for pregnant women to consult with a qualified reflexologist who has experience working with pregnant women before undergoing reflexology treatment. Reflexology should be used as a complementary therapy and should not replace medical care during pregnancy and childbirth.

Preparing for Labor with Reflexology: A Holistic Approach to Childbirth

Preparing for labor is an important part of pregnancy, and reflexology can be a beneficial tool to help women prepare both physically and emotionally for childbirth.

Here's how reflexology can support women as they prepare for labor:

1. Hormonal Balance: Reflexology helps to balance hormones, including oxytocin, which is important for stimulating contractions during labor. By stimulating reflex points associated with hormonal balance, reflexologists can help support the body's natural processes leading up to labor.

2. Pelvic Alignment: Reflexology can help promote pelvic alignment by stimulating reflex points associated with the pelvis and lower back. This can help ensure that the pelvis is properly aligned for childbirth, which can help facilitate a smoother labor process.

3. Relaxation and Stress Reduction: Reflexology promotes relaxation and reduces stress, which can be beneficial as women prepare for labor. By inducing a state of deep relaxation, reflexologists can help women feel more calm and prepared for childbirth.

4. Pain Management: Reflexology can help manage pain and discomfort during labor by stimulating reflex points associated with pain relief. This can help women cope with the intensity of contractions and promote a more comfortable labor experience.

5. Energy Balancing: Reflexology helps to balance the body's energy levels, which can be important during labor. By stimulating reflex points associated with energy levels, reflexologists can help women maintain their stamina and endurance during labor.

6. Emotional Support: Reflexology can provide emotional support as women prepare for labor. By promoting relaxation and reducing anxiety, reflexologists can help women feel more confident and mentally prepared for childbirth.

7. Labor Induction: In some cases, reflexology can be used to help induce labor naturally. By stimulating certain reflex points, reflexologists can help stimulate contractions and encourage the onset of labor.

Overall, reflexology can be a valuable tool to help women prepare for labor and childbirth. It is important for pregnant women to consult with a qualified reflexologist who has experience working with pregnant women before undergoing reflexology treatment. Reflexology should be used as a complementary therapy and should not replace medical care during pregnancy and childbirth.

CHAPTER 9

Reflexology Techniques for Labor Induction: A Natural Approach to Stimulating Contractions

Reflexology can be used as a natural and gentle method to help induce labor when a pregnancy has reached full term and the expectant mother is ready for childbirth. Reflexologists focus on specific reflex points that are believed to stimulate contractions and encourage the onset of labor.

Here are some reflexology techniques that may be used for labor induction:

1. Uterus Reflex Point: Reflexologists focus on stimulating the reflex point for the uterus, which is located on the inside of the heel. By applying firm pressure to this point, reflexologists aim to stimulate contractions and promote the onset of labor.

2. Pituitary Gland Reflex Point: The pituitary gland plays a role in regulating hormones, including oxytocin, which is responsible for stimulating contractions. Reflexologists target the reflex point for the pituitary gland, which is located on the big toe, to help promote hormonal balance and encourage labor.

3. Ovary Reflex Point: The reflex points for the ovaries are located on the outer edge of the foot, near the ankle. Stimulating these points can help promote hormonal balance and support the body as it prepares for labor.

4. Kidney Reflex Points: The kidneys play a role in eliminating waste products from the body, and stimulating the kidney reflex points, located on the inner edge of the foot, near the arch, can help promote detoxification and reduce fluid retention, which can contribute to labor induction.

5. Pelvic Area Reflex Points: Reflexologists target reflex points that correspond to the pelvic area to help promote relaxation and prepare the body for childbirth. By stimulating these points, reflexologists can help support the natural progression of labor.

6. Ankle and Calf Reflex Points: Reflexologists may also target reflex points on the ankles and calves to help stimulate circulation and promote the flow of energy throughout the body, which can help support the onset of labor.

It's important to note that while reflexology can be used as a complementary therapy for labor induction, it should always be done by a qualified reflexologist who has experience working with pregnant women. Pregnant women should also consult with their healthcare provider before undergoing reflexology or any other complementary therapy for labor induction.

Reflexology for Pain Relief During Labor: Supporting Comfort and Relaxation

Reflexology can be a valuable tool to help manage pain and discomfort during labor. By targeting specific reflex points on the feet, hands, or ears, reflexologists can help stimulate the body's natural pain relief mechanisms and promote relaxation, which can be beneficial during labor.

Here's how reflexology can help with pain relief during labor:

1. Pain Relief Reflex Points: Reflexologists focus on stimulating reflex points that are associated with pain relief, such as the spine, head, and neck reflex points. By applying pressure to these points, reflexologists can help reduce pain and discomfort during labor.

2. Endorphin Release: Reflexology stimulates the release of endorphins, which are the body's natural painkillers. By promoting the release of endorphins, reflexologists can help reduce pain and promote a sense of well-being during labor.

3. Relaxation Response: Reflexology promotes relaxation by activating the parasympathetic nervous system, which helps reduce stress and tension in the body. By inducing a state of deep relaxation, reflexologists can help women cope with the intensity of contractions and promote a more comfortable labor experience.

4. Hormonal Balance: Reflexology helps to balance hormones, including oxytocin, which is important for stimulating contractions and promoting relaxation during labor. By stimulating reflex points associated with hormonal balance, reflexologists can help support the body's natural processes during labor.

5. Energy Balancing: Reflexology helps to balance the body's energy levels, which can be important during labor. By stimulating reflex points associated with energy levels, reflexologists can help women maintain their stamina and endurance during labor.

6. Emotional Support: Reflexology can provide emotional support during labor by promoting relaxation and reducing anxiety. By helping women feel more calm and centered, reflexologists can help them cope with the emotional challenges of labor.

Overall, reflexology can be a valuable tool to help manage pain and discomfort during labor. It is important for pregnant women to consult with a qualified reflexologist who has experience working with pregnant women before undergoing reflexology treatment. Reflexology should be used as a complementary therapy and should not replace medical care during labor.

CHAPTER 10

Postnatal Reflexology: Supporting Recovery and Well-being After Childbirth

Postnatal reflexology can be a beneficial therapy for new mothers as they recover from childbirth and adjust to the demands of caring for a newborn. Reflexology can help support the body's natural healing processes, promote relaxation, and alleviate common postnatal issues.

Here's how postnatal reflexology can benefit new mothers:

1. Hormonal Balance: Reflexology can help balance hormones, including prolactin (responsible for milk production) and oxytocin (responsible for uterine contractions and bonding). Balancing these hormones can support breastfeeding and emotional well-being.

2. Stress Reduction: Reflexology promotes relaxation and reduces stress, which is important for new mothers who may be experiencing sleep deprivation and adjusting to the demands of caring for a newborn.

3. Pain Relief: Reflexology can help relieve post nasal discomfort, such as back pain, pelvic pain, and sore muscles, by targeting reflex points associated with pain relief and relaxation.

4. Uterine Involution: Reflexology can help promote uterine involution, the process by which the uterus returns to its pre-pregnancy size, by stimulating reflex points associated with the uterus and reproductive organs.

5. Postnatal Depression: Reflexology can help support emotional well-being and reduce symptoms of postnatal depression by promoting relaxation, reducing stress, and balancing hormones.

6. Energy Balancing: Reflexology helps to balance the body's energy levels, which can be important for new mothers who may be feeling fatigued and overwhelmed.

7. Breast Health: Reflexology can help support breast health and lactation by stimulating reflex points associated with the breasts and lactation.

8. Digestive Health: Reflexology can help support digestive health, which may be disrupted postnatally due to hormonal changes and stress.

Postnatal reflexology sessions are typically gentle and focused on promoting relaxation and well-being. It's important for new mothers to communicate with their reflexologist about their specific needs and concerns. Reflexology should be used as a complementary therapy and should not replace medical care postnatally.

Benefits of Postpartum Reflexology: Supporting Recovery and Well-being After Childbirth

Postpartum reflexology can offer a range of benefits for new mothers as they navigate the physical and emotional changes that come with childbirth.

Here are some key benefits of postpartum reflexology:

1. Hormonal Balance: Reflexology can help balance hormones such as prolactin and oxytocin, which are important for breastfeeding and bonding with the baby. Balancing these hormones can also help regulate mood and reduce the risk of postpartum depression.

2. Pain Relief: Reflexology can help relieve postpartum pain and discomfort, such as back pain, pelvic pain, and sore muscles, by stimulating reflex points associated with pain relief and relaxation.

3. Stress Reduction: Reflexology promotes relaxation and reduces stress, which is important for new mothers who may be experiencing sleep deprivation and adjusting to the demands of caring for a newborn.

4. Uterine Involution: Reflexology can help promote uterine involution, the process by which the uterus returns to its pre-pregnancy size, by stimulating reflex points associated with the uterus and reproductive organs.

5. Improved Sleep: Reflexology can help improve sleep quality and reduce insomnia, which are common issues for new mothers.

6. Increased Energy: Reflexology helps to balance the body's energy levels, which can help new mothers feel more energized and better able to cope with the demands of caring for a newborn.

7. Relaxation and Emotional Well-being: Reflexology promotes relaxation and reduces anxiety, which can help improve overall emotional well-being and reduce the risk of postpartum depression.

8. Breast Health: Reflexology can help support breast health and lactation by stimulating reflex points associated with the breasts and lactation.

9. Digestive Health: Reflexology can help support digestive health, which may be disrupted postnatally due to hormonal changes and stress.

10. Bonding: Reflexology can help promote bonding between mother and baby by promoting relaxation and reducing stress, allowing for more positive interactions between mother and baby.

Overall, postpartum reflexology can be a valuable tool to help new mothers recover from childbirth and adjust to the demands of caring for a newborn. It is important for new mothers to consult with a qualified reflexologist who has experience working with postpartum women before undergoing reflexology treatment. Reflexology should be used as a complementary therapy and should not replace medical care postnatally.

Reflexology for Postpartum Recovery and Healing: Nurturing the Mother's Body and Mind

Reflexology can play a significant role in the postpartum recovery process, offering support for the body's natural healing mechanisms and promoting overall well-being.

Here's how reflexology can aid in postpartum recovery and healing:

1. Hormonal Balance: Reflexology can help balance hormones, including prolactin and oxytocin, which are crucial for breastfeeding and bonding with the baby. Hormonal balance can also support emotional well-being and reduce the risk of postpartum depression.

2. Pain Relief: Reflexology can alleviate postpartum discomfort, such as back pain, pelvic pain, and sore muscles, by targeting reflex points associated with pain relief and relaxation.

3. Stress Reduction: Postpartum reflexology promotes relaxation and reduces stress, which is essential for new mothers adjusting to their new role and managing the demands of caring for a newborn.

4. Uterine Involution: Reflexology can stimulate reflex points associated with the uterus and reproductive organs, supporting the natural process of uterine involution, where the uterus returns to its pre-pregnancy size.

5. Improved Sleep: Reflexology can improve sleep quality and reduce insomnia, common challenges for new mothers.

6. Energy Restoration: By balancing the body's energy levels, reflexology helps new mothers feel more energized and better able to cope with the demands of motherhood.

7. Emotional Support: Reflexology promotes relaxation and reduces anxiety, fostering emotional well-being and reducing the risk of postpartum depression.

8. Breast Health: Reflexology can support breast health and lactation by stimulating reflex points associated with the breasts and milk production.

9. Digestive Health: Reflexology can support digestive health, which may be disrupted postnatally due to hormonal changes and stress.

10. Overall Healing: Reflexology nurtures the body and mind, aiding in overall healing and recovery after childbirth.

Postpartum reflexology sessions are typically gentle and tailored to the individual needs of the mother. It's important for new mothers to communicate with their reflexologist about their specific concerns and comfort levels. Reflexology should complement, not replace, medical care during the postpartum period.

Reflexology for Postpartum Depression: Supporting Emotional Well-being

Postpartum depression (PPD) can significantly impact a new mother's emotional well-being, making it challenging to cope with the demands of caring for a newborn. Reflexology can be a supportive therapy for women experiencing PPD, offering a natural approach to promoting relaxation and emotional balance.

Here's how reflexology can help with postpartum depression:

1. Hormonal Balance: Reflexology can help balance hormones, including cortisol and serotonin, which play a role in mood regulation. By stimulating reflex points associated with hormonal balance, reflexologists can help support emotional well-being.

2. Stress Reduction: Reflexology promotes relaxation and reduces stress, which can be beneficial for women experiencing PPD. By inducing a state of deep relaxation, reflexologists can help women cope with the challenges of PPD and promote a sense of calm.

3. Emotional Release: Reflexology can help release emotional tension and promote a sense of well-being. By stimulating reflex points associated with emotional release, reflexologists can help women process and cope with their feelings.

4. Sleep Improvement: Reflexology can help improve sleep quality, which is often disrupted in women with PPD. By promoting relaxation and reducing anxiety, reflexologists can help women achieve a more restful sleep, which can improve mood and overall well-being.

5. Energy Balancing: Reflexology helps to balance the body's energy levels, which can be important for women with PPD who may feel fatigued and lacking in energy. By stimulating reflex points associated with energy levels, reflexologists can help women feel more energized and motivated.

6. Self-care and Nurturing: Reflexology provides an opportunity for self-care and nurturing, which can be empowering for women with PPD. By taking time for themselves and receiving gentle, nurturing touch, women can feel supported and cared for during a challenging time.

It's important for women experiencing PPD to consult with a qualified reflexologist who has experience working with emotional issues. Reflexology should be used as a complementary therapy and should not replace medical care for PPD. Women with PPD should also seek support from healthcare providers and mental health professionals.

CHAPTER 11

Partner Reflexology Techniques and Support During Pregnancy

Reflexology can be a wonderful way for partners to support each other during pregnancy. While professional reflexology is typically performed by trained practitioners, there are simple techniques partners can use at home to provide comfort and relaxation.

Here are some partner reflexology techniques and support tips for pregnancy:

1. Foot Massage: Gently massaging the feet can help relax the body and alleviate tension. Focus on the heels, arches, and balls of the feet, using gentle pressure and circular motions.

2. Ankle Rotation: Gently rotate each ankle in a circular motion to help improve circulation and reduce swelling in the feet and ankles.

3. Hand Massage: Massaging the hands can also be soothing. Focus on the palms, fingers, and the area between the thumb and index finger.

4. Shoulder and Neck Massage: Use gentle pressure and circular motions to massage the shoulders and neck, which can help relieve tension and promote relaxation.

5. Lower Back Massage: Massaging the lower back can help alleviate back pain and discomfort. Use gentle pressure and circular motions, focusing on the muscles on either side of the spine.

6. Breathing Exercises: Practice deep breathing exercises together to promote relaxation and reduce stress. Encourage your partner to take slow, deep breaths in through the nose and out through the mouth.

7. Emotional Support: Offer your partner emotional support and reassurance. Pregnancy can be a challenging time, and knowing that you are there for them can make a big difference.

8. Encouragement: Encourage your partner to listen to their body and take breaks when needed. Offer to help with household chores or other tasks to reduce their stress and workload.

9. Communication: Keep the lines of communication open and encourage your partner to express their feelings and concerns. Being able to talk openly can help reduce anxiety and stress.

10. Education: Educate yourself about pregnancy and childbirth so you can better understand what your partner is going through. Attend prenatal appointments and childbirth classes together to show your support.

Partner reflexology techniques and support can help strengthen your bond as a couple and provide comfort and relaxation during pregnancy. Always consult with a healthcare provider before trying any new therapies or techniques during pregnancy.

How Partners Can Support Each Other Through Reflexology During Pregnancy

Partners can play a crucial role in supporting each other through pregnancy, and reflexology can be a valuable tool for providing comfort and relaxation.

Here's how partners can support each other through reflexology during pregnancy:

1. Foot Massage: Gentle foot massages can help reduce swelling and discomfort in the feet and ankles. Partners can use their thumbs to apply gentle pressure to the arches and heels of the feet, moving in circular motions.

2. Hand Massage: Massaging the hands can help relieve tension and promote relaxation. Partners can use their thumbs to apply gentle pressure to the palms and fingers, focusing on areas that feel tense.

3. Back Massage: Back massages can help alleviate back pain and discomfort. Partners can use their hands to apply gentle pressure to the lower back, moving in circular motions or using long, sweeping strokes.

4. Shoulder and Neck Massage: Massaging the shoulders and neck can help reduce tension and promote relaxation. Partners can use their fingertips to apply gentle pressure to the shoulders and neck, moving in circular motions.

5. Breathing Exercises: Partners can support each other through breathing exercises, which can help reduce stress and promote relaxation. Partners can practice deep breathing together, focusing on inhaling deeply through the nose and exhaling slowly through the mouth.

6. Communication: Open and honest communication is key to supporting each other through pregnancy. Partners should listen to each other's needs and concerns and be willing to provide emotional support.

7. Encouragement: Partners should encourage each other to take breaks when needed and listen to their bodies. Pregnancy can be physically and emotionally challenging, and partners should be supportive and understanding.

8. Education: Partners can educate themselves about pregnancy and childbirth to better understand what their partner is going through. This can help partners provide more effective support and care.

9. Professional Help: Partners can also support each other by encouraging professional help if needed. If either partner is experiencing severe stress, anxiety, or depression, it's important to seek help from a healthcare professional.

By using reflexology techniques and providing emotional support, partners can help each other navigate the ups and downs of pregnancy and create a strong foundation for their growing family.

Reflexology Techniques for Partners to Learn During Pregnancy

Learning basic reflexology techniques can empower partners to provide effective support and relief during pregnancy.

Here are some simple techniques partners can learn:

1. **Foot Reflexology:** Gently massage the entire foot using the thumb, starting from the heel and moving towards the toes. Apply pressure to specific points on the foot associated with relaxation and pain relief, such as the solar plexus point (beneath the ball of the foot) and the pelvic reflex point (on the inside edge of the foot).

2. Hand Reflexology: Massage the hands using the thumb, focusing on the palm and fingers. Apply pressure to points associated with stress relief and relaxation, such as the adrenal gland reflex point (on the thumb pad) and the diaphragm reflex point (on the middle of the palm).

3. Back Reflexology: Use the hands to apply gentle pressure to the lower back, focusing on areas that feel tense or sore. Use circular motions or long, sweeping strokes to help alleviate back pain and promote relaxation.

4. Shoulder and Neck Reflexology: Massage the shoulders and neck using the fingertips, applying gentle pressure in circular motions. Focus on areas that feel tight or tense to help relieve tension and promote relaxation.

5. Breathing Techniques: Practice deep breathing exercises together, focusing on inhaling deeply through the nose and exhaling slowly through the mouth. This can help reduce stress and promote relaxation for both partners.

6. Communication: Maintain open and honest communication throughout the reflexology session. Encourage your partner to communicate any discomfort or areas that need more attention.

7. Relaxation Techniques: Use soft music, dim lighting, and comfortable pillows to create a relaxing environment for the reflexology session. Encourage your partner to close their eyes and focus on deep breathing to enhance relaxation.

8. Educational Resources: Consider taking a reflexology class together or reading books on reflexology to deepen your understanding of the techniques and their benefits.

By learning these basic reflexology techniques, partners can provide effective support and relief during pregnancy, creating a deeper bond and enhancing the overall pregnancy experience.

Reflexology for Bonding and Relaxation During Pregnancy

Reflexology can be a powerful tool for enhancing bonding and relaxation between partners during pregnancy. By focusing on specific reflex points on the feet and hands, partners can create a sense of connection and promote deep relaxation.

Here's how reflexology can be used for bonding and relaxation during pregnancy:

1. Foot Reflexology: Sit comfortably facing each other, with one partner's feet resting in the other's lap. Gently massage the feet using the thumbs, applying pressure to specific points associated with relaxation and bonding. Use long, sweeping strokes to promote relaxation and stimulate circulation.

2. Hand Reflexology: Hold hands and massage each other's hands using the thumbs, focusing on the palms and fingers. Apply gentle pressure to points associated with stress relief and relaxation, such as the solar plexus point (beneath the ball of the thumb) and the heart reflex point (in the center of the palm).

3. Breathing Exercises: Practice deep breathing together, synchronizing your breath and focusing on inhaling deeply through the nose and exhaling slowly through the mouth. This can help create a sense of unity and relaxation between partners.

4. Communication: Use the reflexology session as an opportunity to communicate openly and honestly with each other. Share your thoughts, feelings, and concerns, and listen attentively to each other's needs.

5. Mindfulness: Encourage each other to be present in the moment and focus on the sensations of the reflexology session. This can help deepen your connection and promote relaxation.

6. Visualization: During the reflexology session, visualize a peaceful and positive experience together. Imagine yourselves bonding with your baby and creating a loving and nurturing environment for your growing family.

7. Relaxation Techniques: Use soft music, dim lighting, and comfortable pillows to create a soothing environment for the reflexology session. Encourage each other to relax deeply and let go of any tension or stress.

By incorporating reflexology into your pregnancy routine, you can enhance bonding and relaxation between partners, creating a positive and nurturing environment for both mother and baby.

CHAPTER 12

Self-Care Reflexology Techniques for Pregnancy

Self-care reflexology techniques can be a valuable tool for pregnant women to promote relaxation, reduce stress, and alleviate common pregnancy discomforts.

Here are some simple techniques that can be done at home:

1. Foot Reflexology: Sit comfortably and place a tennis ball or massage ball under one foot. Roll the ball gently under your foot, applying pressure to different areas. Focus on the heel, arch, and ball of the foot to help relieve tension and promote relaxation.

2. Hand Reflexology: Massage your hands using your thumb, focusing on the palms and fingers. Apply gentle pressure to points associated with stress relief and relaxation, such as the solar plexus point (beneath the ball of the thumb) and the heart reflex point (in the center of the palm).

3. Ear Reflexology: Gently massage your ears using your fingertips, focusing on the earlobes, outer edges, and behind the ears. This can help stimulate relaxation and promote a sense of well-being.

4. Breathing Exercises: Practice deep breathing exercises to help reduce stress and promote relaxation. Inhale deeply through your nose, hold for a few seconds, and exhale slowly through your mouth. Repeat several times to help calm your mind and body.

5. Visualization: Close your eyes and visualize a peaceful and calming scene, such as a beach or a garden. Imagine yourself surrounded by love and positivity, and allow yourself to relax deeply into the visualization.

6. Foot Soak: Fill a basin with warm water and add a few drops of essential oil, such as lavender or chamomile. Soak your feet for 10-15 minutes, allowing the warm water to relax your muscles and promote circulation.

7. Massage: Gently massage your abdomen using circular motions, starting from the lower abdomen and moving upwards towards the ribs. This can help relieve tension and promote relaxation in the abdominal muscles.

8. Hydration: Drink plenty of water throughout the day to stay hydrated and help flush out toxins from your body. Hydration is important for overall health and well-being during pregnancy.

These self-care reflexology techniques can be incorporated into your daily routine to help promote relaxation and well-being during pregnancy. Remember to listen to your body and adjust the pressure and intensity of the techniques to suit your comfort level.

Self-Reflexology Techniques for Pregnancy Wellness

Self-reflexology is a wonderful way for pregnant women to support their well-being, reduce stress, and alleviate discomforts associated with pregnancy.

Here are some simple techniques you can try at home:

1. Foot Reflexology: Sit in a comfortable position and rest one foot on your opposite knee. Use your thumb to apply gentle pressure to the base of your big toe, which is connected to your pituitary gland and can help regulate hormone levels. Massage in a circular motion for a few minutes on each foot.

2. Hand Reflexology: Massage your hands by applying pressure to the area between your thumb and index finger. This is believed to stimulate the release of endorphins, which can help relieve pain and promote relaxation. You can also massage the base of your fingers, which corresponds to the head and neck area.

3. Ear Reflexology: Gently massage your ears by rubbing them between your thumb and index finger. Pay attention to the outer edges of your ears, which correspond to your spine and can help relieve back pain. You can also gently tug on your earlobes to promote relaxation.

4. Breathing Techniques: Practice deep breathing exercises to help calm your mind and relax your body. Inhale slowly through your nose, hold for a few seconds, and exhale through your mouth. Repeat several times, focusing on relaxing your body with each breath.

5. Aromatherapy: Use essential oils like lavender or chamomile to enhance your self-reflexology session. Place a few drops of oil on your palms, rub them together, and inhale deeply. The soothing scent can help promote relaxation and reduce stress.

6. Visualization: Close your eyes and visualize a peaceful scene, such as a beach or a forest. Imagine yourself surrounded by calmness and serenity. Visualizing positive images can help reduce stress and promote relaxation.

7. Hydration: Drink plenty of water throughout the day to stay hydrated and help flush out toxins. Proper hydration is important for overall health and can help alleviate common pregnancy discomforts.

8. Rest and Relaxation: Take time to rest and relax during your pregnancy. Listen to your body and give yourself permission to slow down and take care of yourself.

These self-reflexology techniques can be a valuable addition to your pregnancy wellness routine. However, it's important to consult with your healthcare provider before trying any new therapies, especially if you have any underlying health conditions or concerns.

Reflexology Techniques for Stress Relief and Relaxation

Reflexology offers effective techniques for stress relief and relaxation, promoting a sense of calm and well-being.

Here are some reflexology techniques you can try for stress relief:

1. Foot Reflexology:

- Sit comfortably and remove your shoes.

- Use your thumbs to apply gentle pressure to the reflex points on your feet associated with relaxation, such as the solar plexus point (beneath the ball of your foot) and the adrenal gland reflex point (on the top of your foot, just below the base of your toes).

- Massage in a circular motion, starting from the heels and working towards the toes.

- Focus on deep breathing as you massage your feet, inhaling slowly through your nose and exhaling through your mouth to promote relaxation.

2. Hand Reflexology:

- Sit comfortably and rest your hands on your lap.

- Use your thumb to apply gentle pressure to the reflex points on your hands associated with relaxation, such as the solar plexus point (on the palm, just below the base of your thumb) and the heart reflex point (in the center of your palm).

- Massage in a circular motion, starting from the center of your palm and working towards the edges.

- Focus on deep breathing as you massage your hands, inhaling slowly through your nose and exhaling through your mouth to promote relaxation.

3. Ear Reflexology:

- Gently massage your ears between your thumb and index finger, starting from the earlobes and working towards the outer edges.
- Pay attention to the reflex points on your ears associated with relaxation, such as the brain reflex point (on the outer edge of your ear) and the adrenal gland reflex point (on the inner edge of your ear).
- Massage in a circular motion to stimulate the reflex points and promote relaxation.

4. Breathing Exercises:

- Practice deep breathing exercises to help calm your mind and body.
- Inhale slowly through your nose, counting to four.
- Hold your breath for a few seconds.

- Exhale slowly through your mouth, counting to four.
- Repeat several times, focusing on relaxing your body with each breath.

5. Visualization:

- Close your eyes and visualize a peaceful scene, such as a beach or a forest.
- Imagine yourself surrounded by calmness and serenity.
- Visualizing positive images can help reduce stress and promote relaxation.

Incorporate these reflexology techniques into your daily routine to help relieve stress and promote relaxation. Remember to listen to your body and adjust the pressure and intensity of the techniques to suit your comfort level.

Reflexology for Emotional Well-being

Reflexology can be a powerful tool for promoting emotional well-being, helping to reduce stress, anxiety, and depression. By stimulating specific reflex points on the feet, hands, and ears, reflexology can help balance the body's energy flow and promote a sense of calm and relaxation.

Here's how reflexology can support emotional well-being:

1. Stress Reduction: Reflexology can help reduce stress by promoting relaxation and reducing tension in the body. By stimulating reflex points associated with the adrenal glands and the solar plexus, reflexology can help regulate the body's stress response and promote a sense of calm.

2. Anxiety Relief: Reflexology can help relieve anxiety by promoting relaxation and reducing the body's response to stress. By stimulating reflex points associated with the nervous system and the brain, reflexology can help calm the mind and reduce feelings of anxiety.

3. Mood Enhancement: Reflexology can help enhance mood by stimulating the release of endorphins, the body's natural feel-good hormones. By stimulating reflex points associated with the pituitary gland and the hypothalamus, reflexology can help regulate mood and promote a sense of well-being.

4. Energy Balancing: Reflexology helps balance the body's energy flow, promoting a sense of balance and harmony. By stimulating reflex points associated with the chakras, reflexology can help restore energy balance and promote emotional well-being.

5. Relaxation: Reflexology induces a state of deep relaxation, which can help reduce anxiety and promote emotional well-being. By stimulating reflex points associated with relaxation, reflexology can help calm the mind and body and promote a sense of peace.

6. Self-awareness: Reflexology can help promote self-awareness by encouraging individuals to tune into their bodies and become more mindful of their emotions. By stimulating reflex points associated with the mind-body connection, reflexology can help individuals become more aware of their emotional state and promote emotional well-being.

7. Holistic Healing: Reflexology is a holistic therapy that addresses the body, mind, and spirit. By promoting balance and harmony within the body, reflexology can help support overall emotional well-being and promote a sense of wholeness.

Incorporating reflexology into your self-care routine can be a valuable way to support your emotional well-being. Whether you practice self-reflexology at home or receive treatments from a professional reflexologist, reflexology can be a powerful tool for promoting emotional health and well-being.

CHAPTER 13

Summary of Key Points: Reflexology for Emotional Well-being

1. Stress Reduction: Reflexology can help reduce stress by promoting relaxation and reducing tension in the body.

2. Anxiety Relief: Reflexology can help relieve anxiety by calming the mind and reducing the body's response to stress.

3. Mood Enhancement: Reflexology can enhance mood by stimulating the release of feel-good hormones.

4. Energy Balancing: Reflexology helps balance the body's energy flow, promoting a sense of balance and harmony.

5. Relaxation: Reflexology induces deep relaxation, which can help reduce anxiety and promote emotional well-being.

6. Self-awareness: Reflexology can promote self-awareness by encouraging individuals to tune into their bodies and emotions.

7. Holistic Healing: Reflexology is a holistic therapy that addresses the body, mind, and spirit, promoting overall emotional well-being.

Incorporating reflexology into your self-care routine can be a valuable way to support your emotional well-being and promote a sense of peace and balance in your life.

Reflexology is not just a physical therapy but also a holistic approach to well-being that can have profound effects on your emotional health. By stimulating specific points on the feet, hands, and ears, reflexology can help reduce stress, anxiety, and depression, promoting a sense of calm and relaxation. Whether you practice self-reflexology at home or seek treatment from a professional reflexologist, incorporating reflexology into your routine can be a powerful tool for promoting emotional well-being. Remember to listen to your body and adjust the techniques to suit your comfort level. With regular practice, reflexology can help you achieve a greater sense of balance, harmony, and emotional well-being in your life.

Glossary of Reflexology Terms

1. Reflexology: A holistic therapy that involves applying pressure to specific points on the feet, hands, and ears to promote relaxation, reduce stress, and stimulate healing in the body.

2. Reflex Points: Areas on the feet, hands, and ears that correspond to specific organs, glands, and other parts of the body. Stimulating these points is believed to promote healing and balance in the corresponding areas of the body.

3. Adrenal Glands: Endocrine glands located on top of the kidneys that produce hormones involved in the body's stress response. Reflexology can help balance the function of the adrenal glands, promoting relaxation and reducing stress.

4. Solar Plexus: A complex network of nerves located in the abdomen that plays a role in the body's stress response. Stimulating the solar plexus reflex point is believed to help regulate the body's stress response and promote relaxation.

5. Endorphins: Natural chemicals produced by the body that act as painkillers and mood enhancers. Reflexology can stimulate the release of endorphins, promoting a sense of well-being and reducing pain.

6. Pituitary Gland: An endocrine gland located at the base of the brain that regulates many bodily functions, including growth, metabolism, and stress response. Reflexology can help balance the function of the pituitary gland, promoting hormonal balance and emotional well-being.

7. Hypothalamus: A region of the brain that links the nervous system to the endocrine system and regulates many bodily functions, including body temperature, hunger, and emotions. Reflexology can help balance the function of the hypothalamus, promoting emotional well-being.

8. Chakras: Energy centers in the body that are believed to correspond to different aspects of physical, emotional, and spiritual health. Reflexology can help balance the chakras, promoting overall health and well-being.

9. Self-awareness: The ability to tune into one's own thoughts, feelings, and sensations. Reflexology can promote self-awareness by encouraging individuals to pay attention to their bodies and emotions.

10. Holistic Healing: An approach to health and wellness that considers the whole person, including physical, emotional, and spiritual aspects. Reflexology is a holistic therapy that aims to promote balance and harmony in the body, mind, and spirit.

CONCLUSION

As you reach the end of "Maternity Reflexology Compendium ," you have embarked on a journey of self-discovery, empowerment, and wellness. Throughout this book, we have explored the art and science of reflexology as a powerful tool for enhancing your pregnancy experience.

Empowerment Through Knowledge: One of the key themes of this book has been empowerment through knowledge. By understanding the principles of reflexology and how it can benefit you during pregnancy, you have gained a deeper insight into your body's natural healing abilities. Armed with this knowledge, you are better equipped to take charge of your well-being and make informed choices that support your health and the health of your baby.

Nurturing Your Pregnancy Journey: Pregnancy is a journey like no other, filled with its own unique joys and challenges. Through the practice of reflexology, you have learned how to nurture yourself and your baby, easing discomforts, preparing for labor, and promoting healing and recovery postpartum. Reflexology has not only provided physical relief but also offered you a space for relaxation, connection, and mindfulness during this special time in your life.

Looking Ahead: As you continue your journey into motherhood, remember that reflexology can be a lifelong companion, supporting you through the various stages of motherhood and beyond.

Whether you are navigating the challenges of early motherhood or simply seeking a moment of relaxation and rejuvenation, reflexology can continue to be a valuable tool in your self-care arsenal.

Final Thoughts: As you close the pages of "Maternity Reflexology Compendium ," I encourage you to continue exploring the world of reflexology and its many benefits. Whether you choose to practice reflexology on yourself, seek out a professional reflexologist, or simply incorporate some of the principles of reflexology into your daily life, know that you are taking positive steps towards enhancing your health and well-being.

I invite you to order your copy and order for a friend or relative of "Maternity Reflexology

Compendium " today and embark on a journey of wellness and empowerment. May this book serve as a guide and companion on your path to a happy, healthy, and fulfilling pregnancy journey.

www.ingramcontent.com/pod-product-compliance
Lightning Source LLC
Chambersburg PA
CBHW051612250726
48653CB00004BA/1473